My Cycling Journal: A Diary For Cyclists To Log And Track Their Rides

Dubreck World Publishing

Copyright

'My Cycling Journal: A Diary For Cyclists To Log And Track Their Rides'

First published in August 2021 by Dubreck World Publishing
Printed and bound by Lulu Press
Distributed by Lulu Press

Copyright © 2021 Dubreck World Publishing, Hampshire, UK

All rights reserved. No part of this publication may be reproduced, stored in a retrieval system, or transmitted, in any form or by any means, without the prior permission in writing of the publisher, not be otherwise circulated in any form other than that in which it is published.

ISBN-13: 978-1-326-55832-1
First Edition

DUBRECK WORLD PUBLISHING

If found, please return to

_____

My Bicycle Information

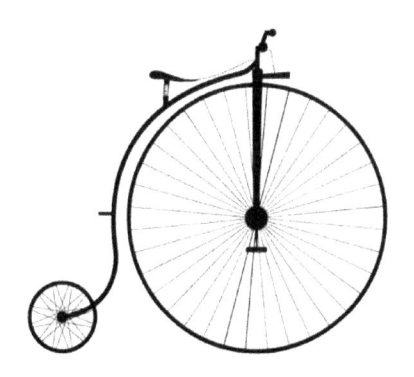

Year:
_____

Make:
_____

Model:
_____

My Cycling Summary

Date	Place	Distance
JANUARY		
1st Jan		
2nd Jan		
3rd Jan		
4th Jan		
5th Jan		
6th Jan		
7th Jan		
8th Jan		
9th Jan		
10th Jan		
11th Jan		
12th Jan		
13th Jan		
14th Jan		
15th Jan		
16th Jan		
17th Jan		
18th Jan		
19th Jan		
20th Jan		
21st Jan		
22nd Jan		
23rd Jan		

24th Jan		
25th Jan		
26th Jan		
27th Jan		
28th Jan		
29th Jan		
30th Jan		
31st Jan		
FEBRUARY		
1st Feb		
2nd Feb		
3rd Feb		
4th Feb		
5th Feb		
6th Feb		
7th Feb		
8th Feb		
9th Feb		
10th Feb		
11th Feb		
12th Feb		
13th Feb		
14th Feb		
15th Feb		
16th Feb		
17th Feb		
18th Feb		

19th Feb		
20th Feb		
21st Feb		
22nd Feb		
23rd Feb		
24th Feb		
25th Feb		
26th Feb		
27th Feb		
28th Feb		
29th Feb		
MARCH		
1st Mar		
2nd Mar		
3rd Mar		
4th Mar		
5th Mar		
6th Mar		
7th Mar		
8th Mar		
9th Mar		
10th Mar		
11th Mar		
12th Mar		
13th Mar		
14th Mar		
15th Mar		

16th Mar		
17th Mar		
18th Mar		
19th Mar		
20th Mar		
21st Mar		
22nd Mar		
23rd Mar		
24th Mar		
25th Mar		
26th Mar		
27th Mar		
28th Mar		
29th Mar		
30th Mar		
31st Mar		
APRIL		
1st Apr		
2nd Apr		
3rd Apr		
4th Apr		
5th Apr		
6th Apr		
7th Apr		
8th Apr		
9th Apr		
10th Apr		

11th Apr		
12th Apr		
13th Apr		
14th Apr		
15th Apr		
16th Apr		
17th Apr		
18th Apr		
19th Apr		
20th Apr		
21st Apr		
22nd Apr		
23rd Apr		
24th Apr		
25th Apr		
26th Apr		
27th Apr		
28th Apr		
29th Apr		
30th Apr		
MAY		
1st May		
2nd May		
3rd May		
4th May		
5th May		
6th May		

7th May		
8th May		
9th May		
10th May		
11th May		
12th May		
13th May		
14th May		
15th May		
16th May		
17th May		
18th May		
19th May		
20th May		
21st May		
22nd May		
23rd May		
24th May		
25th May		
26th May		
27th May		
28th May		
29th May		
30th May		
31st May		
JUNE		
1st June		

2nd June		
3rd June		
4th June		
5th June		
6th June		
7th June		
8th June		
9th June		
10th June		
11th June		
12th June		
13th June		
14th June		
15th June		
16th June		
17th June		
18th June		
19th June		
20th June		
21st June		
22nd June		
23rd June		
24th June		
25th June		
26th June		
27th June		
28th June		

29th June		
30th June		
JULY		
1st July		
2nd July		
3rd July		
4th July		
5th July		
6th July		
7th July		
8th July		
9th July		
10th July		
11th July		
12th July		
13th July		
14th July		
15th July		
16th July		
17th July		
18th July		
19th July		
20th July		
21st July		
22nd July		
23rd July		
24th July		

25th July		
26th July		
27th July		
28th July		
29th July		
30th July		
31st July		
AUGUST		
1st Aug		
2nd Aug		
3rd Aug		
4th Aug		
5th Aug		
6th Aug		
7th Aug		
8th Aug		
9th Aug		
10th Aug		
11th Aug		
12th Aug		
13th Aug		
14th Aug		
15th Aug		
16th Aug		
17th Aug		
18th Aug		
19th Aug		

20th Aug		
21st Aug		
22nd Aug		
23rd Aug		
24th Aug		
25th Aug		
26th Aug		
27th Aug		
28th Aug		
29th Aug		
30th Aug		
31st Aug		
SEPTEMBER		
1st Sept		
2nd Sept		
3rd Sept		
4th Sept		
5th Sept		
6th Sept		
7th Sept		
8th Sept		
9th Sept		
10th Sept		
11th Sept		
12th Sept		
13th Sept		
14th Sept		

15th Sept		
16th Sept		
17th Sept		
18th Sept		
19th Sept		
20th Sept		
21st Sept		
22nd Sept		
23rd Sept		
24th Sept		
25th Sept		
26th Sept		
27th Sept		
28th Sept		
29th Sept		
30th Sept		
OCTOBER		
1st Oct		
2nd Oct		
3rd Oct		
4th Oct		
5th Oct		
6th Oct		
7th Oct		
8th Oct		
9th Oct		
10th Oct		

11th Oct		
12th Oct		
13th Oct		
14th Oct		
15th Oct		
16th Oct		
17th Oct		
18th Oct		
19th Oct		
20th Oct		
21st Oct		
22nd Oct		
23rd Oct		
24th Oct		
25th Oct		
26th Oct		
27th Oct		
28th Oct		
29th Oct		
30th Oct		
31st Oct		
NOVEMBER		
1st Nov		
2nd Nov		
3rd Nov		
4th Nov		
5th Nov		

6th Nov		
7th Nov		
8th Nov		
9th Nov		
10th Nov		
11th Nov		
12th Nov		
13th Nov		
14th Nov		
15th Nov		
16th Nov		
17th Nov		
18th Nov		
19th Nov		
20th Nov		
21st Nov		
22nd Nov		
23rd Nov		
24th Nov		
25th Nov		
26th Nov		
27th Nov		
28th Nov		
29th Nov		
30th Nov		
DECEMBER		
1st Dec		

2nd Dec		
3rd Dec		
4th Dec		
5th Dec		
6th Dec		
7th Dec		
8th Dec		
9th Dec		
10th Dec		
11th Dec		
12th Dec		
13th Dec		
14th Dec		
15th Dec		
16th Dec		
17th Dec		
18th Dec		
19th Dec		
20th Dec		
21st Dec		
22nd Dec		
23rd Dec		
24th Dec		
25th Dec		
26th Dec		
27th Dec		
28th Dec		

29th Dec		
30th Dec		
31st Dec		

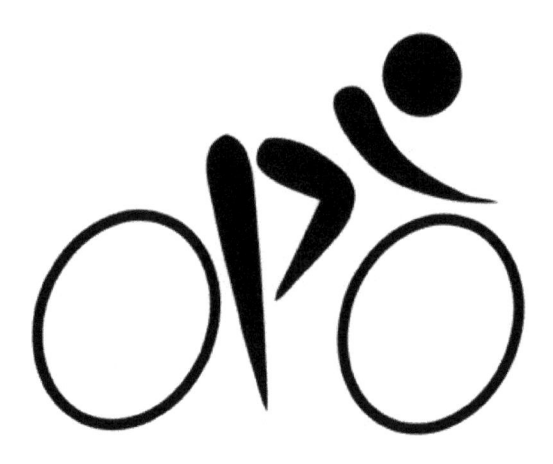

My Cycling Log

"Ride as much or as little, or as long or as short as you feel... but ride"
- Eddy Merckx

Date:	Weather:
Location:	
Trail Conditions:	
Start Time:	End Time:
Duration:	Distance:
Average Speed:	Max Speed:

Date:	Weather:
Location:	
Trail Conditions:	
Start Time:	End Time:
Duration:	Distance:
Average Speed:	Max Speed:

Date:	Weather:
Location:	
Trail Conditions:	
Start Time:	End Time:
Duration:	Distance:
Average Speed:	Max Speed:

Date:	Weather:
Location:	
Trail Conditions:	
Start Time:	End Time:
Duration:	Distance:
Average Speed:	Max Speed:

Notes:

Date:	Weather:
Location:	
Trail Conditions:	
Start Time:	End Time:
Duration:	Distance:
Average Speed:	Max Speed:

Date:	Weather:
Location:	
Trail Conditions:	
Start Time:	End Time:
Duration:	Distance:
Average Speed:	Max Speed:

Date:	Weather:
Location:	
Trail Conditions:	
Start Time:	End Time:
Duration:	Distance:
Average Speed:	Max Speed:

Date:	Weather:
Location:	
Trail Conditions:	
Start Time:	End Time:
Duration:	Distance:
Average Speed:	Max Speed:

Notes:

Date:	Weather:
Location:	
Trail Conditions:	
Start Time:	End Time:
Duration:	Distance:
Average Speed:	Max Speed:

Date:	Weather:
Location:	
Trail Conditions:	
Start Time:	End Time:
Duration:	Distance:
Average Speed:	Max Speed:

Date:	Weather:
Location:	
Trail Conditions:	
Start Time:	End Time:
Duration:	Distance:
Average Speed:	Max Speed:

Date:	Weather:
Location:	
Trail Conditions:	
Start Time:	End Time:
Duration:	Distance:
Average Speed:	Max Speed:

Notes:

Date:	Weather:
Location:	
Trail Conditions:	
Start Time:	End Time:
Duration:	Distance:
Average Speed:	Max Speed:

Date:	Weather:
Location:	
Trail Conditions:	
Start Time:	End Time:
Duration:	Distance:
Average Speed:	Max Speed:

Date:	Weather:
Location:	
Trail Conditions:	
Start Time:	End Time:
Duration:	Distance:
Average Speed:	Max Speed:

Date:	Weather:
Location:	
Trail Conditions:	
Start Time:	End Time:
Duration:	Distance:
Average Speed:	Max Speed:

Notes:

Date:	Weather:
Location:	
Trail Conditions:	
Start Time:	End Time:
Duration:	Distance:
Average Speed:	Max Speed:

Date:	Weather:
Location:	
Trail Conditions:	
Start Time:	End Time:
Duration:	Distance:
Average Speed:	Max Speed:

Date:	Weather:
Location:	
Trail Conditions:	
Start Time:	End Time:
Duration:	Distance:
Average Speed:	Max Speed:

Date:	Weather:
Location:	
Trail Conditions:	
Start Time:	End Time:
Duration:	Distance:
Average Speed:	Max Speed:

Notes:

Date:	Weather:
Location:	
Trail Conditions:	
Start Time:	End Time:
Duration:	Distance:
Average Speed:	Max Speed:

Date:	Weather:
Location:	
Trail Conditions:	
Start Time:	End Time:
Duration:	Distance:
Average Speed:	Max Speed:

Date:	Weather:
Location:	
Trail Conditions:	
Start Time:	End Time:
Duration:	Distance:
Average Speed:	Max Speed:

Date:	Weather:
Location:	
Trail Conditions:	
Start Time:	End Time:
Duration:	Distance:
Average Speed:	Max Speed:

Notes:

Date:	Weather:
Location:	
Trail Conditions:	
Start Time:	End Time:
Duration:	Distance:
Average Speed:	Max Speed:

Date:	Weather:
Location:	
Trail Conditions:	
Start Time:	End Time:
Duration:	Distance:
Average Speed:	Max Speed:

Date:	Weather:
Location:	
Trail Conditions:	
Start Time:	End Time:
Duration:	Distance:
Average Speed:	Max Speed:

Date:	Weather:
Location:	
Trail Conditions:	
Start Time:	End Time:
Duration:	Distance:
Average Speed:	Max Speed:

Notes:

Date:	Weather:
Location:	
Trail Conditions:	
Start Time:	End Time:
Duration:	Distance:
Average Speed:	Max Speed:

Date:	Weather:
Location:	
Trail Conditions:	
Start Time:	End Time:
Duration:	Distance:
Average Speed:	Max Speed:

Date:	Weather:
Location:	
Trail Conditions:	
Start Time:	End Time:
Duration:	Distance:
Average Speed:	Max Speed:

Date:	Weather:
Location:	
Trail Conditions:	
Start Time:	End Time:
Duration:	Distance:
Average Speed:	Max Speed:

Notes:

Date:	Weather:
Location:	
Trail Conditions:	
Start Time:	End Time:
Duration:	Distance:
Average Speed:	Max Speed:

Date:	Weather:
Location:	
Trail Conditions:	
Start Time:	End Time:
Duration:	Distance:
Average Speed:	Max Speed:

Date:	Weather:
Location:	
Trail Conditions:	
Start Time:	End Time:
Duration:	Distance:
Average Speed:	Max Speed:

Date:	Weather:
Location:	
Trail Conditions:	
Start Time:	End Time:
Duration:	Distance:
Average Speed:	Max Speed:

Notes:

Date:	Weather:
Location:	
Trail Conditions:	
Start Time:	End Time:
Duration:	Distance:
Average Speed:	Max Speed:

Date:	Weather:
Location:	
Trail Conditions:	
Start Time:	End Time:
Duration:	Distance:
Average Speed:	Max Speed:

Date:	Weather:
Location:	
Trail Conditions:	
Start Time:	End Time:
Duration:	Distance:
Average Speed:	Max Speed:

Date:	Weather:
Location:	
Trail Conditions:	
Start Time:	End Time:
Duration:	Distance:
Average Speed:	Max Speed:

Notes:

Date:	Weather:
Location:	
Trail Conditions:	
Start Time:	End Time:
Duration:	Distance:
Average Speed:	Max Speed:

Date:	Weather:
Location:	
Trail Conditions:	
Start Time:	End Time:
Duration:	Distance:
Average Speed:	Max Speed:

Date:	Weather:
Location:	
Trail Conditions:	
Start Time:	End Time:
Duration:	Distance:
Average Speed:	Max Speed:

Date:	Weather:
Location:	
Trail Conditions:	
Start Time:	End Time:
Duration:	Distance:
Average Speed:	Max Speed:

Notes:

Date:	Weather:
Location:	
Trail Conditions:	
Start Time:	End Time:
Duration:	Distance:
Average Speed:	Max Speed:

Date:	Weather:
Location:	
Trail Conditions:	
Start Time:	End Time:
Duration:	Distance:
Average Speed:	Max Speed:

Date:	Weather:
Location:	
Trail Conditions:	
Start Time:	End Time:
Duration:	Distance:
Average Speed:	Max Speed:

Date:	Weather:
Location:	
Trail Conditions:	
Start Time:	End Time:
Duration:	Distance:
Average Speed:	Max Speed:

Notes:

Date:	Weather:
Location:	
Trail Conditions:	
Start Time:	End Time:
Duration:	Distance:
Average Speed:	Max Speed:

Date:	Weather:
Location:	
Trail Conditions:	
Start Time:	End Time:
Duration:	Distance:
Average Speed:	Max Speed:

Date:	Weather:
Location:	
Trail Conditions:	
Start Time:	End Time:
Duration:	Distance:
Average Speed:	Max Speed:

Date:	Weather:
Location:	
Trail Conditions:	
Start Time:	End Time:
Duration:	Distance:
Average Speed:	Max Speed:

Notes:

Date:	Weather:
Location:	
Trail Conditions:	
Start Time:	End Time:
Duration:	Distance:
Average Speed:	Max Speed:

Date:	Weather:
Location:	
Trail Conditions:	
Start Time:	End Time:
Duration:	Distance:
Average Speed:	Max Speed:

Date:	Weather:
Location:	
Trail Conditions:	
Start Time:	End Time:
Duration:	Distance:
Average Speed:	Max Speed:

Date:	Weather:
Location:	
Trail Conditions:	
Start Time:	End Time:
Duration:	Distance:
Average Speed:	Max Speed:

Notes:

Date:	Weather:
Location:	
Trail Conditions:	
Start Time:	End Time:
Duration:	Distance:
Average Speed:	Max Speed:

Date:	Weather:
Location:	
Trail Conditions:	
Start Time:	End Time:
Duration:	Distance:
Average Speed:	Max Speed:

Date:	Weather:
Location:	
Trail Conditions:	
Start Time:	End Time:
Duration:	Distance:
Average Speed:	Max Speed:

Date:	Weather:
Location:	
Trail Conditions:	
Start Time:	End Time:
Duration:	Distance:
Average Speed:	Max Speed:

Notes:

Date:	Weather:
Location:	
Trail Conditions:	
Start Time:	End Time:
Duration:	Distance:
Average Speed:	Max Speed:

Date:	Weather:
Location:	
Trail Conditions:	
Start Time:	End Time:
Duration:	Distance:
Average Speed:	Max Speed:

Date:	Weather:
Location:	
Trail Conditions:	
Start Time:	End Time:
Duration:	Distance:
Average Speed:	Max Speed:

Date:	Weather:
Location:	
Trail Conditions:	
Start Time:	End Time:
Duration:	Distance:
Average Speed:	Max Speed:

Notes:

Date:	Weather:
Location:	
Trail Conditions:	
Start Time:	End Time:
Duration:	Distance:
Average Speed:	Max Speed:

Date:	Weather:
Location:	
Trail Conditions:	
Start Time:	End Time:
Duration:	Distance:
Average Speed:	Max Speed:

Date:	Weather:
Location:	
Trail Conditions:	
Start Time:	End Time:
Duration:	Distance:
Average Speed:	Max Speed:

Date:	Weather:
Location:	
Trail Conditions:	
Start Time:	End Time:
Duration:	Distance:
Average Speed:	Max Speed:

Notes:

Date:	Weather:
Location:	
Trail Conditions:	
Start Time:	End Time:
Duration:	Distance:
Average Speed:	Max Speed:

Date:	Weather:
Location:	
Trail Conditions:	
Start Time:	End Time:
Duration:	Distance:
Average Speed:	Max Speed:

Date:	Weather:
Location:	
Trail Conditions:	
Start Time:	End Time:
Duration:	Distance:
Average Speed:	Max Speed:

Date:	Weather:
Location:	
Trail Conditions:	
Start Time:	End Time:
Duration:	Distance:
Average Speed:	Max Speed:

Notes:

Date:	Weather:
Location:	
Trail Conditions:	
Start Time:	End Time:
Duration:	Distance:
Average Speed:	Max Speed:

Date:	Weather:
Location:	
Trail Conditions:	
Start Time:	End Time:
Duration:	Distance:
Average Speed:	Max Speed:

Date:	Weather:
Location:	
Trail Conditions:	
Start Time:	End Time:
Duration:	Distance:
Average Speed:	Max Speed:

Date:	Weather:
Location:	
Trail Conditions:	
Start Time:	End Time:
Duration:	Distance:
Average Speed:	Max Speed:

Notes:

Date:	Weather:
Location:	
Trail Conditions:	
Start Time:	End Time:
Duration:	Distance:
Average Speed:	Max Speed:

Date:	Weather:
Location:	
Trail Conditions:	
Start Time:	End Time:
Duration:	Distance:
Average Speed:	Max Speed:

Date:	Weather:
Location:	
Trail Conditions:	
Start Time:	End Time:
Duration:	Distance:
Average Speed:	Max Speed:

Date:	Weather:
Location:	
Trail Conditions:	
Start Time:	End Time:
Duration:	Distance:
Average Speed:	Max Speed:

Notes:

Date:	Weather:
Location:	
Trail Conditions:	
Start Time:	End Time:
Duration:	Distance:
Average Speed:	Max Speed:

Date:	Weather:
Location:	
Trail Conditions:	
Start Time:	End Time:
Duration:	Distance:
Average Speed:	Max Speed:

Date:	Weather:
Location:	
Trail Conditions:	
Start Time:	End Time:
Duration:	Distance:
Average Speed:	Max Speed:

Date:	Weather:
Location:	
Trail Conditions:	
Start Time:	End Time:
Duration:	Distance:
Average Speed:	Max Speed:

Notes:

Date:	Weather:
Location:	
Trail Conditions:	
Start Time:	End Time:
Duration:	Distance:
Average Speed:	Max Speed:

Date:	Weather:
Location:	
Trail Conditions:	
Start Time:	End Time:
Duration:	Distance:
Average Speed:	Max Speed:

Date:	Weather:
Location:	
Trail Conditions:	
Start Time:	End Time:
Duration:	Distance:
Average Speed:	Max Speed:

Date:	Weather:
Location:	
Trail Conditions:	
Start Time:	End Time:
Duration:	Distance:
Average Speed:	Max Speed:

Notes:

Date:	Weather:
Location:	
Trail Conditions:	
Start Time:	End Time:
Duration:	Distance:
Average Speed:	Max Speed:

Date:	Weather:
Location:	
Trail Conditions:	
Start Time:	End Time:
Duration:	Distance:
Average Speed:	Max Speed:

Date:	Weather:
Location:	
Trail Conditions:	
Start Time:	End Time:
Duration:	Distance:
Average Speed:	Max Speed:

Date:	Weather:
Location:	
Trail Conditions:	
Start Time:	End Time:
Duration:	Distance:
Average Speed:	Max Speed:

Notes:

Date:	Weather:
Location:	
Trail Conditions:	
Start Time:	End Time:
Duration:	Distance:
Average Speed:	Max Speed:

Date:	Weather:
Location:	
Trail Conditions:	
Start Time:	End Time:
Duration:	Distance:
Average Speed:	Max Speed:

Date:	Weather:
Location:	
Trail Conditions:	
Start Time:	End Time:
Duration:	Distance:
Average Speed:	Max Speed:

Date:	Weather:
Location:	
Trail Conditions:	
Start Time:	End Time:
Duration:	Distance:
Average Speed:	Max Speed:

Notes:

Date:	Weather:
Location:	
Trail Conditions:	
Start Time:	End Time:
Duration:	Distance:
Average Speed:	Max Speed:

Date:	Weather:
Location:	
Trail Conditions:	
Start Time:	End Time:
Duration:	Distance:
Average Speed:	Max Speed:

Date:	Weather:
Location:	
Trail Conditions:	
Start Time:	End Time:
Duration:	Distance:
Average Speed:	Max Speed:

Date:	Weather:
Location:	
Trail Conditions:	
Start Time:	End Time:
Duration:	Distance:
Average Speed:	Max Speed:

Notes:

Date:	Weather:
Location:	
Trail Conditions:	
Start Time:	End Time:
Duration:	Distance:
Average Speed:	Max Speed:

Date:	Weather:
Location:	
Trail Conditions:	
Start Time:	End Time:
Duration:	Distance:
Average Speed:	Max Speed:

Date:	Weather:
Location:	
Trail Conditions:	
Start Time:	End Time:
Duration:	Distance:
Average Speed:	Max Speed:

Date:	Weather:
Location:	
Trail Conditions:	
Start Time:	End Time:
Duration:	Distance:
Average Speed:	Max Speed:

Notes:

Date:	Weather:
Location:	
Trail Conditions:	
Start Time:	End Time:
Duration:	Distance:
Average Speed:	Max Speed:

Date:	Weather:
Location:	
Trail Conditions:	
Start Time:	End Time:
Duration:	Distance:
Average Speed:	Max Speed:

Date:	Weather:
Location:	
Trail Conditions:	
Start Time:	End Time:
Duration:	Distance:
Average Speed:	Max Speed:

Date:	Weather:
Location:	
Trail Conditions:	
Start Time:	End Time:
Duration:	Distance:
Average Speed:	Max Speed:

Notes:

Date:	Weather:
Location:	
Trail Conditions:	
Start Time:	End Time:
Duration:	Distance:
Average Speed:	Max Speed:

Date:	Weather:
Location:	
Trail Conditions:	
Start Time:	End Time:
Duration:	Distance:
Average Speed:	Max Speed:

Date:	Weather:
Location:	
Trail Conditions:	
Start Time:	End Time:
Duration:	Distance:
Average Speed:	Max Speed:

Date:	Weather:
Location:	
Trail Conditions:	
Start Time:	End Time:
Duration:	Distance:
Average Speed:	Max Speed:

Notes:

Date:	Weather:
Location:	
Trail Conditions:	
Start Time:	End Time:
Duration:	Distance:
Average Speed:	Max Speed:

Date:	Weather:
Location:	
Trail Conditions:	
Start Time:	End Time:
Duration:	Distance:
Average Speed:	Max Speed:

Date:	Weather:
Location:	
Trail Conditions:	
Start Time:	End Time:
Duration:	Distance:
Average Speed:	Max Speed:

Date:	Weather:
Location:	
Trail Conditions:	
Start Time:	End Time:
Duration:	Distance:
Average Speed:	Max Speed:

Notes:

Date:	Weather:
Location:	
Trail Conditions:	
Start Time:	End Time:
Duration:	Distance:
Average Speed:	Max Speed:

Date:	Weather:
Location:	
Trail Conditions:	
Start Time:	End Time:
Duration:	Distance:
Average Speed:	Max Speed:

Date:	Weather:
Location:	
Trail Conditions:	
Start Time:	End Time:
Duration:	Distance:
Average Speed:	Max Speed:

Date:	Weather:
Location:	
Trail Conditions:	
Start Time:	End Time:
Duration:	Distance:
Average Speed:	Max Speed:

Notes:

Date:	Weather:
Location:	
Trail Conditions:	
Start Time:	End Time:
Duration:	Distance:
Average Speed:	Max Speed:

Date:	Weather:
Location:	
Trail Conditions:	
Start Time:	End Time:
Duration:	Distance:
Average Speed:	Max Speed:

Date:	Weather:
Location:	
Trail Conditions:	
Start Time:	End Time:
Duration:	Distance:
Average Speed:	Max Speed:

Date:	Weather:
Location:	
Trail Conditions:	
Start Time:	End Time:
Duration:	Distance:
Average Speed:	Max Speed:

Notes:

Date:	Weather:
Location:	
Trail Conditions:	
Start Time:	End Time:
Duration:	Distance:
Average Speed:	Max Speed:

Date:	Weather:
Location:	
Trail Conditions:	
Start Time:	End Time:
Duration:	Distance:
Average Speed:	Max Speed:

Date:	Weather:
Location:	
Trail Conditions:	
Start Time:	End Time:
Duration:	Distance:
Average Speed:	Max Speed:

Date:	Weather:
Location:	
Trail Conditions:	
Start Time:	End Time:
Duration:	Distance:
Average Speed:	Max Speed:

Notes:

Date:	Weather:
Location:	
Trail Conditions:	
Start Time:	End Time:
Duration:	Distance:
Average Speed:	Max Speed:

Date:	Weather:
Location:	
Trail Conditions:	
Start Time:	End Time:
Duration:	Distance:
Average Speed:	Max Speed:

Date:	Weather:
Location:	
Trail Conditions:	
Start Time:	End Time:
Duration:	Distance:
Average Speed:	Max Speed:

Date:	Weather:
Location:	
Trail Conditions:	
Start Time:	End Time:
Duration:	Distance:
Average Speed:	Max Speed:

Notes:

Date:	Weather:
Location:	
Trail Conditions:	
Start Time:	End Time:
Duration:	Distance:
Average Speed:	Max Speed:

Date:	Weather:
Location:	
Trail Conditions:	
Start Time:	End Time:
Duration:	Distance:
Average Speed:	Max Speed:

Date:	Weather:
Location:	
Trail Conditions:	
Start Time:	End Time:
Duration:	Distance:
Average Speed:	Max Speed:

Date:	Weather:
Location:	
Trail Conditions:	
Start Time:	End Time:
Duration:	Distance:
Average Speed:	Max Speed:

Notes:

Date:	Weather:
Location:	
Trail Conditions:	
Start Time:	End Time:
Duration:	Distance:
Average Speed:	Max Speed:

Date:	Weather:
Location:	
Trail Conditions:	
Start Time:	End Time:
Duration:	Distance:
Average Speed:	Max Speed:

Date:	Weather:
Location:	
Trail Conditions:	
Start Time:	End Time:
Duration:	Distance:
Average Speed:	Max Speed:

Date:	Weather:
Location:	
Trail Conditions:	
Start Time:	End Time:
Duration:	Distance:
Average Speed:	Max Speed:

Notes:

Date:	Weather:
Location:	
Trail Conditions:	
Start Time:	End Time:
Duration:	Distance:
Average Speed:	Max Speed:

Date:	Weather:
Location:	
Trail Conditions:	
Start Time:	End Time:
Duration:	Distance:
Average Speed:	Max Speed:

Date:	Weather:
Location:	
Trail Conditions:	
Start Time:	End Time:
Duration:	Distance:
Average Speed:	Max Speed:

Date:	Weather:
Location:	
Trail Conditions:	
Start Time:	End Time:
Duration:	Distance:
Average Speed:	Max Speed:

Notes:

Date:	Weather:
Location:	
Trail Conditions:	
Start Time:	End Time:
Duration:	Distance:
Average Speed:	Max Speed:

Date:	Weather:
Location:	
Trail Conditions:	
Start Time:	End Time:
Duration:	Distance:
Average Speed:	Max Speed:

Date:	Weather:
Location:	
Trail Conditions:	
Start Time:	End Time:
Duration:	Distance:
Average Speed:	Max Speed:

Date:	Weather:
Location:	
Trail Conditions:	
Start Time:	End Time:
Duration:	Distance:
Average Speed:	Max Speed:

Notes:

Date:	Weather:
Location:	
Trail Conditions:	
Start Time:	End Time:
Duration:	Distance:
Average Speed:	Max Speed:

Date:	Weather:
Location:	
Trail Conditions:	
Start Time:	End Time:
Duration:	Distance:
Average Speed:	Max Speed:

Date:	Weather:
Location:	
Trail Conditions:	
Start Time:	End Time:
Duration:	Distance:
Average Speed:	Max Speed:

Date:	Weather:
Location:	
Trail Conditions:	
Start Time:	End Time:
Duration:	Distance:
Average Speed:	Max Speed:

Notes:

Date:	Weather:
Location:	
Trail Conditions:	
Start Time:	End Time:
Duration:	Distance:
Average Speed:	Max Speed:

Date:	Weather:
Location:	
Trail Conditions:	
Start Time:	End Time:
Duration:	Distance:
Average Speed:	Max Speed:

Date:	Weather:
Location:	
Trail Conditions:	
Start Time:	End Time:
Duration:	Distance:
Average Speed:	Max Speed:

Date:	Weather:
Location:	
Trail Conditions:	
Start Time:	End Time:
Duration:	Distance:
Average Speed:	Max Speed:

Notes:

Date:	Weather:
Location:	
Trail Conditions:	
Start Time:	End Time:
Duration:	Distance:
Average Speed:	Max Speed:

Date:	Weather:
Location:	
Trail Conditions:	
Start Time:	End Time:
Duration:	Distance:
Average Speed:	Max Speed:

Date:	Weather:
Location:	
Trail Conditions:	
Start Time:	End Time:
Duration:	Distance:
Average Speed:	Max Speed:

Date:	Weather:
Location:	
Trail Conditions:	
Start Time:	End Time:
Duration:	Distance:
Average Speed:	Max Speed:

Notes:

Date:	Weather:
Location:	
Trail Conditions:	
Start Time:	End Time:
Duration:	Distance:
Average Speed:	Max Speed:

Date:	Weather:
Location:	
Trail Conditions:	
Start Time:	End Time:
Duration:	Distance:
Average Speed:	Max Speed:

Date:	Weather:
Location:	
Trail Conditions:	
Start Time:	End Time:
Duration:	Distance:
Average Speed:	Max Speed:

Date:	Weather:
Location:	
Trail Conditions:	
Start Time:	End Time:
Duration:	Distance:
Average Speed:	Max Speed:

Notes:

Date:	Weather:
Location:	
Trail Conditions:	
Start Time:	End Time:
Duration:	Distance:
Average Speed:	Max Speed:

Date:	Weather:
Location:	
Trail Conditions:	
Start Time:	End Time:
Duration:	Distance:
Average Speed:	Max Speed:

Date:	Weather:
Location:	
Trail Conditions:	
Start Time:	End Time:
Duration:	Distance:
Average Speed:	Max Speed:

Date:	Weather:
Location:	
Trail Conditions:	
Start Time:	End Time:
Duration:	Distance:
Average Speed:	Max Speed:

Notes:

Date:	Weather:
Location:	
Trail Conditions:	
Start Time:	End Time:
Duration:	Distance:
Average Speed:	Max Speed:

Date:	Weather:
Location:	
Trail Conditions:	
Start Time:	End Time:
Duration:	Distance:
Average Speed:	Max Speed:

Date:	Weather:
Location:	
Trail Conditions:	
Start Time:	End Time:
Duration:	Distance:
Average Speed:	Max Speed:

Date:	Weather:
Location:	
Trail Conditions:	
Start Time:	End Time:
Duration:	Distance:
Average Speed:	Max Speed:

Notes:

Date:	Weather:
Location:	
Trail Conditions:	
Start Time:	End Time:
Duration:	Distance:
Average Speed:	Max Speed:

Date:	Weather:
Location:	
Trail Conditions:	
Start Time:	End Time:
Duration:	Distance:
Average Speed:	Max Speed:

Date:	Weather:
Location:	
Trail Conditions:	
Start Time:	End Time:
Duration:	Distance:
Average Speed:	Max Speed:

Date:	Weather:
Location:	
Trail Conditions:	
Start Time:	End Time:
Duration:	Distance:
Average Speed:	Max Speed:

Notes:

Date:	Weather:
Location:	
Trail Conditions:	
Start Time:	End Time:
Duration:	Distance:
Average Speed:	Max Speed:

Date:	Weather:
Location:	
Trail Conditions:	
Start Time:	End Time:
Duration:	Distance:
Average Speed:	Max Speed:

Date:	Weather:
Location:	
Trail Conditions:	
Start Time:	End Time:
Duration:	Distance:
Average Speed:	Max Speed:

Date:	Weather:
Location:	
Trail Conditions:	
Start Time:	End Time:
Duration:	Distance:
Average Speed:	Max Speed:

Notes:

Date:	Weather:
Location:	
Trail Conditions:	
Start Time:	End Time:
Duration:	Distance:
Average Speed:	Max Speed:

Date:	Weather:
Location:	
Trail Conditions:	
Start Time:	End Time:
Duration:	Distance:
Average Speed:	Max Speed:

Date:	Weather:
Location:	
Trail Conditions:	
Start Time:	End Time:
Duration:	Distance:
Average Speed:	Max Speed:

Date:	Weather:
Location:	
Trail Conditions:	
Start Time:	End Time:
Duration:	Distance:
Average Speed:	Max Speed:

Notes:

Date:	Weather:
Location:	
Trail Conditions:	
Start Time:	End Time:
Duration:	Distance:
Average Speed:	Max Speed:

Date:	Weather:
Location:	
Trail Conditions:	
Start Time:	End Time:
Duration:	Distance:
Average Speed:	Max Speed:

Date:	Weather:
Location:	
Trail Conditions:	
Start Time:	End Time:
Duration:	Distance:
Average Speed:	Max Speed:

Date:	Weather:
Location:	
Trail Conditions:	
Start Time:	End Time:
Duration:	Distance:
Average Speed:	Max Speed:

Notes:

Date:	Weather:
Location:	
Trail Conditions:	
Start Time:	End Time:
Duration:	Distance:
Average Speed:	Max Speed:

Date:	Weather:
Location:	
Trail Conditions:	
Start Time:	End Time:
Duration:	Distance:
Average Speed:	Max Speed:

Date:	Weather:
Location:	
Trail Conditions:	
Start Time:	End Time:
Duration:	Distance:
Average Speed:	Max Speed:

Date:	Weather:
Location:	
Trail Conditions:	
Start Time:	End Time:
Duration:	Distance:
Average Speed:	Max Speed:

Notes:

Date:	Weather:
Location:	
Trail Conditions:	
Start Time:	End Time:
Duration:	Distance:
Average Speed:	Max Speed:

Date:	Weather:
Location:	
Trail Conditions:	
Start Time:	End Time:
Duration:	Distance:
Average Speed:	Max Speed:

Date:	Weather:
Location:	
Trail Conditions:	
Start Time:	End Time:
Duration:	Distance:
Average Speed:	Max Speed:

Date:	Weather:
Location:	
Trail Conditions:	
Start Time:	End Time:
Duration:	Distance:
Average Speed:	Max Speed:

Notes:

Date:	Weather:
Location:	
Trail Conditions:	
Start Time:	End Time:
Duration:	Distance:
Average Speed:	Max Speed:

Date:	Weather:
Location:	
Trail Conditions:	
Start Time:	End Time:
Duration:	Distance:
Average Speed:	Max Speed:

Date:	Weather:
Location:	
Trail Conditions:	
Start Time:	End Time:
Duration:	Distance:
Average Speed:	Max Speed:

Date:	Weather:
Location:	
Trail Conditions:	
Start Time:	End Time:
Duration:	Distance:
Average Speed:	Max Speed:

Notes:

Date:	Weather:
Location:	
Trail Conditions:	
Start Time:	End Time:
Duration:	Distance:
Average Speed:	Max Speed:

Date:	Weather:
Location:	
Trail Conditions:	
Start Time:	End Time:
Duration:	Distance:
Average Speed:	Max Speed:

Date:	Weather:
Location:	
Trail Conditions:	
Start Time:	End Time:
Duration:	Distance:
Average Speed:	Max Speed:

Date:	Weather:
Location:	
Trail Conditions:	
Start Time:	End Time:
Duration:	Distance:
Average Speed:	Max Speed:

Notes:

Date:	Weather:
Location:	
Trail Conditions:	
Start Time:	End Time:
Duration:	Distance:
Average Speed:	Max Speed:

Date:	Weather:
Location:	
Trail Conditions:	
Start Time:	End Time:
Duration:	Distance:
Average Speed:	Max Speed:

Date:	Weather:
Location:	
Trail Conditions:	
Start Time:	End Time:
Duration:	Distance:
Average Speed:	Max Speed:

Date:	Weather:
Location:	
Trail Conditions:	
Start Time:	End Time:
Duration:	Distance:
Average Speed:	Max Speed:

Notes:

Date:	Weather:
Location:	
Trail Conditions:	
Start Time:	End Time:
Duration:	Distance:
Average Speed:	Max Speed:

Date:	Weather:
Location:	
Trail Conditions:	
Start Time:	End Time:
Duration:	Distance:
Average Speed:	Max Speed:

Date:	Weather:
Location:	
Trail Conditions:	
Start Time:	End Time:
Duration:	Distance:
Average Speed:	Max Speed:

Date:	Weather:
Location:	
Trail Conditions:	
Start Time:	End Time:
Duration:	Distance:
Average Speed:	Max Speed:

Notes:

Date:	Weather:
Location:	
Trail Conditions:	
Start Time:	End Time:
Duration:	Distance:
Average Speed:	Max Speed:

Date:	Weather:
Location:	
Trail Conditions:	
Start Time:	End Time:
Duration:	Distance:
Average Speed:	Max Speed:

Date:	Weather:
Location:	
Trail Conditions:	
Start Time:	End Time:
Duration:	Distance:
Average Speed:	Max Speed:

Date:	Weather:
Location:	
Trail Conditions:	
Start Time:	End Time:
Duration:	Distance:
Average Speed:	Max Speed:

Notes:

Date:	Weather:
Location:	
Trail Conditions:	
Start Time:	End Time:
Duration:	Distance:
Average Speed:	Max Speed:

Date:	Weather:
Location:	
Trail Conditions:	
Start Time:	End Time:
Duration:	Distance:
Average Speed:	Max Speed:

Date:	Weather:
Location:	
Trail Conditions:	
Start Time:	End Time:
Duration:	Distance:
Average Speed:	Max Speed:

Date:	Weather:
Location:	
Trail Conditions:	
Start Time:	End Time:
Duration:	Distance:
Average Speed:	Max Speed:

Notes:

Date:	Weather:
Location:	
Trail Conditions:	
Start Time:	End Time:
Duration:	Distance:
Average Speed:	Max Speed:

Date:	Weather:
Location:	
Trail Conditions:	
Start Time:	End Time:
Duration:	Distance:
Average Speed:	Max Speed:

Date:	Weather:
Location:	
Trail Conditions:	
Start Time:	End Time:
Duration:	Distance:
Average Speed:	Max Speed:

Date:	Weather:
Location:	
Trail Conditions:	
Start Time:	End Time:
Duration:	Distance:
Average Speed:	Max Speed:

Notes:

Date:	Weather:
Location:	
Trail Conditions:	
Start Time:	End Time:
Duration:	Distance:
Average Speed:	Max Speed:

Date:	Weather:
Location:	
Trail Conditions:	
Start Time:	End Time:
Duration:	Distance:
Average Speed:	Max Speed:

Date:	Weather:
Location:	
Trail Conditions:	
Start Time:	End Time:
Duration:	Distance:
Average Speed:	Max Speed:

Date:	Weather:
Location:	
Trail Conditions:	
Start Time:	End Time:
Duration:	Distance:
Average Speed:	Max Speed:

Notes:

Date:	Weather:
Location:	
Trail Conditions:	
Start Time:	End Time:
Duration:	Distance:
Average Speed:	Max Speed:

Date:	Weather:
Location:	
Trail Conditions:	
Start Time:	End Time:
Duration:	Distance:
Average Speed:	Max Speed:

Date:	Weather:
Location:	
Trail Conditions:	
Start Time:	End Time:
Duration:	Distance:
Average Speed:	Max Speed:

Date:	Weather:
Location:	
Trail Conditions:	
Start Time:	End Time:
Duration:	Distance:
Average Speed:	Max Speed:

Notes:

Date:	Weather:
Location:	
Trail Conditions:	
Start Time:	End Time:
Duration:	Distance:
Average Speed:	Max Speed:

Date:	Weather:
Location:	
Trail Conditions:	
Start Time:	End Time:
Duration:	Distance:
Average Speed:	Max Speed:

Date:	Weather:
Location:	
Trail Conditions:	
Start Time:	End Time:
Duration:	Distance:
Average Speed:	Max Speed:

Date:	Weather:
Location:	
Trail Conditions:	
Start Time:	End Time:
Duration:	Distance:
Average Speed:	Max Speed:

Notes:

Date:	Weather:
Location:	
Trail Conditions:	
Start Time:	End Time:
Duration:	Distance:
Average Speed:	Max Speed:

Date:	Weather:
Location:	
Trail Conditions:	
Start Time:	End Time:
Duration:	Distance:
Average Speed:	Max Speed:

Date:	Weather:
Location:	
Trail Conditions:	
Start Time:	End Time:
Duration:	Distance:
Average Speed:	Max Speed:

Date:	Weather:
Location:	
Trail Conditions:	
Start Time:	End Time:
Duration:	Distance:
Average Speed:	Max Speed:

Notes:

Date:	Weather:
Location:	
Trail Conditions:	
Start Time:	End Time:
Duration:	Distance:
Average Speed:	Max Speed:

Date:	Weather:
Location:	
Trail Conditions:	
Start Time:	End Time:
Duration:	Distance:
Average Speed:	Max Speed:

Date:	Weather:
Location:	
Trail Conditions:	
Start Time:	End Time:
Duration:	Distance:
Average Speed:	Max Speed:

Date:	Weather:
Location:	
Trail Conditions:	
Start Time:	End Time:
Duration:	Distance:
Average Speed:	Max Speed:

Notes:

Date:	Weather:
Location:	
Trail Conditions:	
Start Time:	End Time:
Duration:	Distance:
Average Speed:	Max Speed:

Date:	Weather:
Location:	
Trail Conditions:	
Start Time:	End Time:
Duration:	Distance:
Average Speed:	Max Speed:

Date:	Weather:
Location:	
Trail Conditions:	
Start Time:	End Time:
Duration:	Distance:
Average Speed:	Max Speed:

Date:	Weather:
Location:	
Trail Conditions:	
Start Time:	End Time:
Duration:	Distance:
Average Speed:	Max Speed:

Notes:

Date:	Weather:
Location:	
Trail Conditions:	
Start Time:	End Time:
Duration:	Distance:
Average Speed:	Max Speed:

Date:	Weather:
Location:	
Trail Conditions:	
Start Time:	End Time:
Duration:	Distance:
Average Speed:	Max Speed:

Date:	Weather:
Location:	
Trail Conditions:	
Start Time:	End Time:
Duration:	Distance:
Average Speed:	Max Speed:

Date:	Weather:
Location:	
Trail Conditions:	
Start Time:	End Time:
Duration:	Distance:
Average Speed:	Max Speed:

Notes:

Date:	Weather:
Location:	
Trail Conditions:	
Start Time:	End Time:
Duration:	Distance:
Average Speed:	Max Speed:

Date:	Weather:
Location:	
Trail Conditions:	
Start Time:	End Time:
Duration:	Distance:
Average Speed:	Max Speed:

Date:	Weather:
Location:	
Trail Conditions:	
Start Time:	End Time:
Duration:	Distance:
Average Speed:	Max Speed:

Date:	Weather:
Location:	
Trail Conditions:	
Start Time:	End Time:
Duration:	Distance:
Average Speed:	Max Speed:

Notes:

Date:	Weather:
Location:	
Trail Conditions:	
Start Time:	End Time:
Duration:	Distance:
Average Speed:	Max Speed:

Date:	Weather:
Location:	
Trail Conditions:	
Start Time:	End Time:
Duration:	Distance:
Average Speed:	Max Speed:

Date:	Weather:
Location:	
Trail Conditions:	
Start Time:	End Time:
Duration:	Distance:
Average Speed:	Max Speed:

Date:	Weather:
Location:	
Trail Conditions:	
Start Time:	End Time:
Duration:	Distance:
Average Speed:	Max Speed:

Notes:

Date:	Weather:
Location:	
Trail Conditions:	
Start Time:	End Time:
Duration:	Distance:
Average Speed:	Max Speed:

Date:	Weather:
Location:	
Trail Conditions:	
Start Time:	End Time:
Duration:	Distance:
Average Speed:	Max Speed:

Date:	Weather:
Location:	
Trail Conditions:	
Start Time:	End Time:
Duration:	Distance:
Average Speed:	Max Speed:

Date:	Weather:
Location:	
Trail Conditions:	
Start Time:	End Time:
Duration:	Distance:
Average Speed:	Max Speed:

Notes:

Date:	Weather:
Location:	
Trail Conditions:	
Start Time:	End Time:
Duration:	Distance:
Average Speed:	Max Speed:

Date:	Weather:
Location:	
Trail Conditions:	
Start Time:	End Time:
Duration:	Distance:
Average Speed:	Max Speed:

Date:	Weather:
Location:	
Trail Conditions:	
Start Time:	End Time:
Duration:	Distance:
Average Speed:	Max Speed:

Date:	Weather:
Location:	
Trail Conditions:	
Start Time:	End Time:
Duration:	Distance:
Average Speed:	Max Speed:

Notes:

Date:	Weather:
Location:	
Trail Conditions:	
Start Time:	End Time:
Duration:	Distance:
Average Speed:	Max Speed:

Date:	Weather:
Location:	
Trail Conditions:	
Start Time:	End Time:
Duration:	Distance:
Average Speed:	Max Speed:

Date:	Weather:
Location:	
Trail Conditions:	
Start Time:	End Time:
Duration:	Distance:
Average Speed:	Max Speed:

Date:	Weather:
Location:	
Trail Conditions:	
Start Time:	End Time:
Duration:	Distance:
Average Speed:	Max Speed:

Notes:

Date:	Weather:
Location:	
Trail Conditions:	
Start Time:	End Time:
Duration:	Distance:
Average Speed:	Max Speed:

Date:	Weather:
Location:	
Trail Conditions:	
Start Time:	End Time:
Duration:	Distance:
Average Speed:	Max Speed:

Date:	Weather:
Location:	
Trail Conditions:	
Start Time:	End Time:
Duration:	Distance:
Average Speed:	Max Speed:

Date:	Weather:
Location:	
Trail Conditions:	
Start Time:	End Time:
Duration:	Distance:
Average Speed:	Max Speed:

Notes:

Date:	Weather:
Location:	
Trail Conditions:	
Start Time:	End Time:
Duration:	Distance:
Average Speed:	Max Speed:

Date:	Weather:
Location:	
Trail Conditions:	
Start Time:	End Time:
Duration:	Distance:
Average Speed:	Max Speed:

Date:	Weather:
Location:	
Trail Conditions:	
Start Time:	End Time:
Duration:	Distance:
Average Speed:	Max Speed:

Date:	Weather:
Location:	
Trail Conditions:	
Start Time:	End Time:
Duration:	Distance:
Average Speed:	Max Speed:

Notes:

Date:	Weather:
Location:	
Trail Conditions:	
Start Time:	End Time:
Duration:	Distance:
Average Speed:	Max Speed:

Date:	Weather:
Location:	
Trail Conditions:	
Start Time:	End Time:
Duration:	Distance:
Average Speed:	Max Speed:

Date:	Weather:
Location:	
Trail Conditions:	
Start Time:	End Time:
Duration:	Distance:
Average Speed:	Max Speed:

Date:	Weather:
Location:	
Trail Conditions:	
Start Time:	End Time:
Duration:	Distance:
Average Speed:	Max Speed:

Notes:

Date:	Weather:
Location:	
Trail Conditions:	
Start Time:	End Time:
Duration:	Distance:
Average Speed:	Max Speed:

Date:	Weather:
Location:	
Trail Conditions:	
Start Time:	End Time:
Duration:	Distance:
Average Speed:	Max Speed:

Date:	Weather:
Location:	
Trail Conditions:	
Start Time:	End Time:
Duration:	Distance:
Average Speed:	Max Speed:

Date:	Weather:
Location:	
Trail Conditions:	
Start Time:	End Time:
Duration:	Distance:
Average Speed:	Max Speed:

Notes:

Date:	Weather:
Location:	
Trail Conditions:	
Start Time:	End Time:
Duration:	Distance:
Average Speed:	Max Speed:

Date:	Weather:
Location:	
Trail Conditions:	
Start Time:	End Time:
Duration:	Distance:
Average Speed:	Max Speed:

Date:	Weather:
Location:	
Trail Conditions:	
Start Time:	End Time:
Duration:	Distance:
Average Speed:	Max Speed:

Date:	Weather:
Location:	
Trail Conditions:	
Start Time:	End Time:
Duration:	Distance:
Average Speed:	Max Speed:

Notes:

Date:	Weather:
Location:	
Trail Conditions:	
Start Time:	End Time:
Duration:	Distance:
Average Speed:	Max Speed:

Date:	Weather:
Location:	
Trail Conditions:	
Start Time:	End Time:
Duration:	Distance:
Average Speed:	Max Speed:

Date:	Weather:
Location:	
Trail Conditions:	
Start Time:	End Time:
Duration:	Distance:
Average Speed:	Max Speed:

Date:	Weather:
Location:	
Trail Conditions:	
Start Time:	End Time:
Duration:	Distance:
Average Speed:	Max Speed:

Notes:

Date:	Weather:
Location:	
Trail Conditions:	
Start Time:	End Time:
Duration:	Distance:
Average Speed:	Max Speed:

Date:	Weather:
Location:	
Trail Conditions:	
Start Time:	End Time:
Duration:	Distance:
Average Speed:	Max Speed:

Date:	Weather:
Location:	
Trail Conditions:	
Start Time:	End Time:
Duration:	Distance:
Average Speed:	Max Speed:

Date:	Weather:
Location:	
Trail Conditions:	
Start Time:	End Time:
Duration:	Distance:
Average Speed:	Max Speed:

Notes:

Date:	Weather:
Location:	
Trail Conditions:	
Start Time:	End Time:
Duration:	Distance:
Average Speed:	Max Speed:

Date:	Weather:
Location:	
Trail Conditions:	
Start Time:	End Time:
Duration:	Distance:
Average Speed:	Max Speed:

Date:	Weather:
Location:	
Trail Conditions:	
Start Time:	End Time:
Duration:	Distance:
Average Speed:	Max Speed:

Date:	Weather:
Location:	
Trail Conditions:	
Start Time:	End Time:
Duration:	Distance:
Average Speed:	Max Speed:

Notes:

Date:	Weather:
Location:	
Trail Conditions:	
Start Time:	End Time:
Duration:	Distance:
Average Speed:	Max Speed:

Date:	Weather:
Location:	
Trail Conditions:	
Start Time:	End Time:
Duration:	Distance:
Average Speed:	Max Speed:

Date:	Weather:
Location:	
Trail Conditions:	
Start Time:	End Time:
Duration:	Distance:
Average Speed:	Max Speed:

Date:	Weather:
Location:	
Trail Conditions:	
Start Time:	End Time:
Duration:	Distance:
Average Speed:	Max Speed:

Notes:

Date:	Weather:
Location:	
Trail Conditions:	
Start Time:	End Time:
Duration:	Distance:
Average Speed:	Max Speed:

Date:	Weather:
Location:	
Trail Conditions:	
Start Time:	End Time:
Duration:	Distance:
Average Speed:	Max Speed:

Date:	Weather:
Location:	
Trail Conditions:	
Start Time:	End Time:
Duration:	Distance:
Average Speed:	Max Speed:

Date:	Weather:
Location:	
Trail Conditions:	
Start Time:	End Time:
Duration:	Distance:
Average Speed:	Max Speed:

Notes:

Date:	Weather:
Location:	
Trail Conditions:	
Start Time:	End Time:
Duration:	Distance:
Average Speed:	Max Speed:

Date:	Weather:
Location:	
Trail Conditions:	
Start Time:	End Time:
Duration:	Distance:
Average Speed:	Max Speed:

Date:	Weather:
Location:	
Trail Conditions:	
Start Time:	End Time:
Duration:	Distance:
Average Speed:	Max Speed:

Date:	Weather:
Location:	
Trail Conditions:	
Start Time:	End Time:
Duration:	Distance:
Average Speed:	Max Speed:

Notes:

Date:	Weather:
Location:	
Trail Conditions:	
Start Time:	End Time:
Duration:	Distance:
Average Speed:	Max Speed:

Date:	Weather:
Location:	
Trail Conditions:	
Start Time:	End Time:
Duration:	Distance:
Average Speed:	Max Speed:

Date:	Weather:
Location:	
Trail Conditions:	
Start Time:	End Time:
Duration:	Distance:
Average Speed:	Max Speed:

Date:	Weather:
Location:	
Trail Conditions:	
Start Time:	End Time:
Duration:	Distance:
Average Speed:	Max Speed:

Notes:

Date:	Weather:
Location:	
Trail Conditions:	
Start Time:	End Time:
Duration:	Distance:
Average Speed:	Max Speed:

Date:	Weather:
Location:	
Trail Conditions:	
Start Time:	End Time:
Duration:	Distance:
Average Speed:	Max Speed:

Date:	Weather:
Location:	
Trail Conditions:	
Start Time:	End Time:
Duration:	Distance:
Average Speed:	Max Speed:

Date:	Weather:
Location:	
Trail Conditions:	
Start Time:	End Time:
Duration:	Distance:
Average Speed:	Max Speed:

Notes:

Date:	Weather:
Location:	
Trail Conditions:	
Start Time:	End Time:
Duration:	Distance:
Average Speed:	Max Speed:

Date:	Weather:
Location:	
Trail Conditions:	
Start Time:	End Time:
Duration:	Distance:
Average Speed:	Max Speed:

Date:	Weather:
Location:	
Trail Conditions:	
Start Time:	End Time:
Duration:	Distance:
Average Speed:	Max Speed:

Date:	Weather:
Location:	
Trail Conditions:	
Start Time:	End Time:
Duration:	Distance:
Average Speed:	Max Speed:

Notes:

Date:	Weather:
Location:	
Trail Conditions:	
Start Time:	End Time:
Duration:	Distance:
Average Speed:	Max Speed:

Date:	Weather:
Location:	
Trail Conditions:	
Start Time:	End Time:
Duration:	Distance:
Average Speed:	Max Speed:

Date:	Weather:
Location:	
Trail Conditions:	
Start Time:	End Time:
Duration:	Distance:
Average Speed:	Max Speed:

Date:	Weather:
Location:	
Trail Conditions:	
Start Time:	End Time:
Duration:	Distance:
Average Speed:	Max Speed:

Notes:

Date:	Weather:
Location:	
Trail Conditions:	
Start Time:	End Time:
Duration:	Distance:
Average Speed:	Max Speed:

Date:	Weather:
Location:	
Trail Conditions:	
Start Time:	End Time:
Duration:	Distance:
Average Speed:	Max Speed:

Date:	Weather:
Location:	
Trail Conditions:	
Start Time:	End Time:
Duration:	Distance:
Average Speed:	Max Speed:

Date:	Weather:
Location:	
Trail Conditions:	
Start Time:	End Time:
Duration:	Distance:
Average Speed:	Max Speed:

Notes:

Date:	Weather:
Location:	
Trail Conditions:	
Start Time:	End Time:
Duration:	Distance:
Average Speed:	Max Speed:

Date:	Weather:
Location:	
Trail Conditions:	
Start Time:	End Time:
Duration:	Distance:
Average Speed:	Max Speed:

Date:	Weather:
Location:	
Trail Conditions:	
Start Time:	End Time:
Duration:	Distance:
Average Speed:	Max Speed:

Date:	Weather:
Location:	
Trail Conditions:	
Start Time:	End Time:
Duration:	Distance:
Average Speed:	Max Speed:

Notes:

Date:	Weather:
Location:	
Trail Conditions:	
Start Time:	End Time:
Duration:	Distance:
Average Speed:	Max Speed:

Date:	Weather:
Location:	
Trail Conditions:	
Start Time:	End Time:
Duration:	Distance:
Average Speed:	Max Speed:

Date:	Weather:
Location:	
Trail Conditions:	
Start Time:	End Time:
Duration:	Distance:
Average Speed:	Max Speed:

Date:	Weather:
Location:	
Trail Conditions:	
Start Time:	End Time:
Duration:	Distance:
Average Speed:	Max Speed:

Notes:

Date:	Weather:
Location:	
Trail Conditions:	
Start Time:	End Time:
Duration:	Distance:
Average Speed:	Max Speed:

Date:	Weather:
Location:	
Trail Conditions:	
Start Time:	End Time:
Duration:	Distance:
Average Speed:	Max Speed:

Date:	Weather:
Location:	
Trail Conditions:	
Start Time:	End Time:
Duration:	Distance:
Average Speed:	Max Speed:

Date:	Weather:
Location:	
Trail Conditions:	
Start Time:	End Time:
Duration:	Distance:
Average Speed:	Max Speed:

Notes:

Date:	Weather:
Location:	
Trail Conditions:	
Start Time:	End Time:
Duration:	Distance:
Average Speed:	Max Speed:

Date:	Weather:
Location:	
Trail Conditions:	
Start Time:	End Time:
Duration:	Distance:
Average Speed:	Max Speed:

Date:	Weather:
Location:	
Trail Conditions:	
Start Time:	End Time:
Duration:	Distance:
Average Speed:	Max Speed:

Date:	Weather:
Location:	
Trail Conditions:	
Start Time:	End Time:
Duration:	Distance:
Average Speed:	Max Speed:

Notes:

Date:	Weather:
Location:	
Trail Conditions:	
Start Time:	End Time:
Duration:	Distance:
Average Speed:	Max Speed:

Date:	Weather:
Location:	
Trail Conditions:	
Start Time:	End Time:
Duration:	Distance:
Average Speed:	Max Speed:

Date:	Weather:
Location:	
Trail Conditions:	
Start Time:	End Time:
Duration:	Distance:
Average Speed:	Max Speed:

Date:	Weather:
Location:	
Trail Conditions:	
Start Time:	End Time:
Duration:	Distance:
Average Speed:	Max Speed:

Notes:

Date:	Weather:
Location:	
Trail Conditions:	
Start Time:	End Time:
Duration:	Distance:
Average Speed:	Max Speed:

Date:	Weather:
Location:	
Trail Conditions:	
Start Time:	End Time:
Duration:	Distance:
Average Speed:	Max Speed:

Date:	Weather:
Location:	
Trail Conditions:	
Start Time:	End Time:
Duration:	Distance:
Average Speed:	Max Speed:

Date:	Weather:
Location:	
Trail Conditions:	
Start Time:	End Time:
Duration:	Distance:
Average Speed:	Max Speed:

Notes:

Date:	Weather:
Location:	
Trail Conditions:	
Start Time:	End Time:
Duration:	Distance:
Average Speed:	Max Speed:

Date:	Weather:
Location:	
Trail Conditions:	
Start Time:	End Time:
Duration:	Distance:
Average Speed:	Max Speed:

Date:	Weather:
Location:	
Trail Conditions:	
Start Time:	End Time:
Duration:	Distance:
Average Speed:	Max Speed:

Date:	Weather:
Location:	
Trail Conditions:	
Start Time:	End Time:
Duration:	Distance:
Average Speed:	Max Speed:

Notes:

Date:	Weather:
Location:	
Trail Conditions:	
Start Time:	End Time:
Duration:	Distance:
Average Speed:	Max Speed:

Date:	Weather:
Location:	
Trail Conditions:	
Start Time:	End Time:
Duration:	Distance:
Average Speed:	Max Speed:

Date:	Weather:
Location:	
Trail Conditions:	
Start Time:	End Time:
Duration:	Distance:
Average Speed:	Max Speed:

Date:	Weather:
Location:	
Trail Conditions:	
Start Time:	End Time:
Duration:	Distance:
Average Speed:	Max Speed:

Notes:

My Cycling Notes

🚴